# THE SPUR BOOK
## of
## SNORKELLING

# THE SPUR BOOK
## of
## SNORKELLING

by

Terry Brown and Rob Hunter

SPURBOOKS LIMITED

PUBLISHED BY
Spurbooks Ltd
6 Parade Court
Bourne End
Bucks

*The authors and Spurbooks gratefully acknowledge the help of Jerry Hazzard, Director of Coaching, The British Sub-Aqua Club, in the preparation and writing of this book.*

ISBN 0 904978 09 5

Printed by Maund & Irvine Ltd. Tring, Herts.

# CONTENTS

# INTRODUCTION

Venture Guides are written for those who enjoy active leisure pursuits, out of doors, in all weathers and frequently in remote areas. They aim to provide outdoor enthusiasts with information on a wide range of skills with which to expand their activities, without which their pastimes are more risky and less fun.

Venture Guides, therefore, cover such subjects as Map Reading and Compass Work, Knots, Camping, Basic Sailing, and now, Snorkelling. Further books will cover First Aid, Survival Techniques, Weather Lore, and Physical Fitness, all essential skills for the outdoor enthusiast.

## WHY SNORKELLING?

By far the largest part of the earth's surface is covered by water. This fact is often stated, in varying proportions, and the statement usually refers to salt water, the great seas and oceans, ignoring the many lakes, rivers, ponds, reservoirs, streams and canals, which also seam the land in which we live and travel about.

Today, water provides the basis for a whole range of outdoor activities; sailing, power-boating, canoeing, surfing, cruising, natural history, fishing, swimming, and sub-aqua diving. Those who enjoy activities on or in water, are increasingly involved in exploring the life under the surface.

For all those who enjoy water sports, a knowledge of underwater skills and the ability to use simple diving equipment, such as that required for snorkelling, is an extension of their existing activities, and sometimes a very necessary part of their present pursuits.

Yachtsmen and power-craft people, need to dive sometimes, to free a line round the prop, clear a fouled anchor, or just to pick up something lost overboard in shallow water.

Clearing growth from the bottom, or weed around the echo-sounder, are tasks made much easier with the aid of facemask, snorkel tube and fins.

Naturalists can study fish and pond life underwater, easily, with snorkelling gear, while swimmers and fishermen should all be able to dive below the surface of their chosen element.

For those who are, by inclination, interested in sub-aqua diving with an aqualung, a knowledge of snorkelling techniques is an essential part of initial training, and for all these people and the many thousands of holiday snorkellers, this book is written.

## ABOUT THIS BOOK

This is a book about snorkelling. It covers all aspects of swimming in, and diving under, the surface of the water, wearing the three essentials of a facemask, a snorkel tube and fins. It covers the purchase of suitable equipment, tells you where and how to train, and gives you guide-lines on just how good you need to be to snorkel dive successfully. It also covers safety drills, and rescue and resuscitation techniques.

**FIGURE 1**

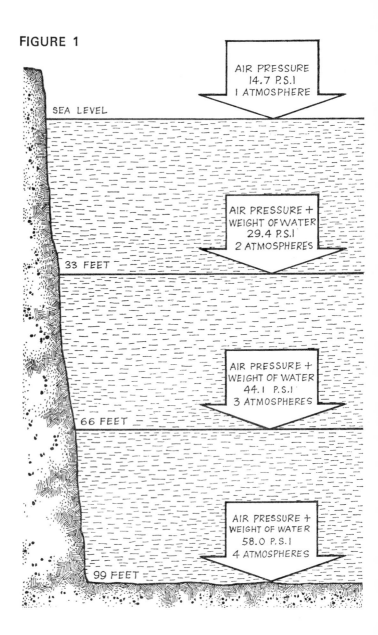

AIR PRESSURE
14.7 P.S.I
1 ATMOSPHERE

SEA LEVEL

AIR PRESSURE +
WEIGHT OF WATER
29.4 P.S.I
2 ATMOSPHERES

33 FEET

AIR PRESSURE +
WEIGHT OF WATER
44.1 P.S.I
3 ATMOSPHERES

66 FEET

AIR PRESSURE +
WEIGHT OF WATER
58.0 P.S.I
4 ATMOSPHERES

99 FEET

It does **NOT** cover aqualung diving, and the drills taught here are not sufficient for anyone to purchase an aqualung and, without further instruction, dive beneath the waves. To learn aqualung diving, you **MUST** have competent training by a good instructor. This is best achieved by joining your local sub-aqua club.

This is a book about snorkelling. By applying the rules herein, and following the instruction carefully, you can, with practice, safely explore the shallow waters of the world beneath the waves, with only your own skill, fitness and commonsense as the limits.

## WHO CAN, AND CANNOT, SNORKEL

Basically, anyone who can swim can go snorkelling.

You must be able to swim. Snorkel divers breathe normal, atmospheric air, and there is no risk of the 'bends', nitrogen narcosis, air embolisms, or other dangers which await aqualung and helmet divers, who are trained to avoid them.

Snorkelling does expose the diver to increases in pressure as he dives deeper, and for this reason people with chronic sinus or ear problems, with heart conditions, or those who suffer from respiratory ailments such as asthma, must be advised to leave it alone, or at least consult their doctor before taking up the sport. Age in itself is no real drawback. Competent swimmers can start snorkelling at about eight years old, and go on virtually for ever.

## PRESSURE; and CLEARING THE EARS

Lest we have alarmed you, let us now explain more about pressure, and put any unreasonable fears to rest before we begin.

Just walking on the surface of the earth puts us all under an **atmospheric pressure** of about 15 lbs per square inch. As we rise up or fall, in an aeroplane for example, this pressure varies, and the effect is most noticeable in the ears. Most people will have experienced discomfort when flying, perhaps with pains in the ears during the descent. Such pain is caused by changes in pressure and is usually eased by swallowing, yawning, or holding the nose and blowing sharply, thus equalizing the pressure in the ears.

The action allows air in the nasal tract to pass through a narrow connecting passage to the middle ear, where it balances the pressure on the outside of the eardrum. At the same time, pressure differences in the sinus cavities of the skull will also be equalised, for these too are connected to the nasal passages.

Underwater, the problem is more acute, for water as an element is much denser than air, and the pressure on the body increases rapidly, so that by 33 ft. it has doubled; 33 ft. of water exerting the same pressure as all the earth's atmosphere. So, at a depth of 33 ft. the body is exposed to a pressure of 30 lbs. per square inch; twice atmospheric pressure. In the same way, at 66 ft. this pressure is three times as much (45 lbs. per sq. inch) (Fig. 1).

It is not very likely that, on the information to be found in this book alone, you will dive to 66 ft. but when skilled at snorkelling you could easily dive to 33 ft. and meet a pressure of two atmospheres. Even at about 10 ft. you will feel pressure and may need to **clear your ears** by pinching the nose and blowing. Your face-mask must have a compensator, so that you are able to pinch your nostrils (Fig. 6, Page 17).

## FIGURE 2

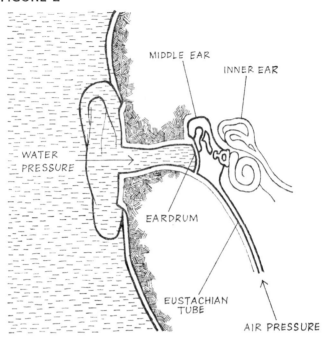

WATER PRESSURE ON THE EARDRUM CAN BE
CLEARED BY PINCHING THE NOSE AND BLOWING

Pressure and the need to compensate for its effects, therefore affects the equipment you buy, and the drills you must learn, as we shall see in future chapters. Once these drills are learnt, and they are really quite simple, there is nothing to worry about.

Because of the effects of increased pressure on the ears and sinuses when diving, anyone suffering from a cold or with a 'stuffy nose' condition, should not go snorkelling until the condition has cleared up. Infected mucus could be forced into the middle ear cavity, or sinus, where it could cause trouble.

## NOSE CLIPS AND EAR PLUGS

It follows from this that you should never wear a nose clip, which prevents you combating "mask squeeze" when pressure forces the mask against the face. Also, you should never wear ear plugs. The pressure may force them into the outer ear passage and do great damage. Some beginners have the belief that nose clips and ear plugs are essential, quite the contrary—with proper equipment, they are totally unnecessary.

# Chapter 1

## SEEING, BREATHING AND MOVING
## UNDERWATER

The facemask is the most wonderful invention. Our instructor, after many years experience of diving, can still recall vividly, the first time he put on a mask and put his face in the water. "It was a wonderland", and that just about sums it up. The facemask is a passport to another world, a looking-glass into a wholly different dimension. With a snorkel tube, through which to breathe air while swimming, face submerged, on the surface, and a pair of fins to help propulsion, you can join the fish in their own element.

The facemask works because, if properly fitted, it excludes the water and provides an air space between your eyes and the water. Your eyes need air space to function efficiently and the mask allows you to see as well beneath the surface as you can above. But you can't see as far. Even the clearest water is denser than air, and the water is frequently clouded, but within the limits of vision you will see objects perfectly. Objects seen underwater appear larger than they really are, and although the brain adjusts to cope with familiar objects, to begin with you can be misled by unusual ones. A tin-can will look normal because you know how big a tin-can ought to look, but a lobster which, underwater looks large enough to feed the family, appears a very small snack, once brought out of the water. So remember that objects underwater appear larger and nearer than they actually are (Fig. 3).

The snorkel tube enables you to breathe while keeping your face under the surface. The tube should be about 12 to 15 inches long at the most. If you get a longer one (if you could find one!) you are only increasing the distance between your lungs and fresh air, and at the same time providing more space for water to fill up when you dive. Water pressure effectively prevents a person from inhaling through a snorkel if the person is deeper than about eighteen inches below the surface.

The final essential item is swim-fins or flippers. These, as is readily apparent, were adapted from webbed frog feet, and must be one of the few items adapted by Man directly from nature, which actually work. Think of all those characters down the Ages, who cast themselves off castle walls wearing artificial birds' wings, and plummeted into the moat! Fins are much simpler than that and highly efficient, especially underwater.

You can add to this **basic equipment** a whole range of accessories, and if you get the snorkelling bug you will probably wish to do so. We will cover a range of accessories later in this book, but before we go any further, let us talk about safety.

FIGURE 3

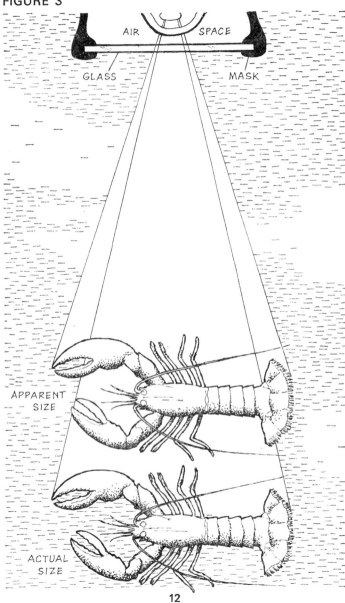

## SAFETY

In all our Venture Guides, we lay stress on safety. There is nothing 'cissy' about playing safe, and nothing 'tough' or 'rugged' about taking chances. You are simply a fool, and if your stupidity leads others to risk their lives in rescue attempts, then you are a dangerous fool. This said and grasped, let us continue by accepting that every activity has its risks, which are in many ways part of the fun, and what you must learn to do is cope with them. There are always a few basic rules which you NEVER break, however experienced you become. The first rule here is:—

1. **NEVER DIVE ALONE.** Always have a partner—or, in sub-aqua parlance, a buddy.

2. **NEVER DIVE UNLESS YOU ARE A COMPETENT SWIMMER.**
   Now here we have a problem, for while many people can swim, not all have passed, or could pass, a swimming test. Most of the approved swimming tests call for the ability to swim 300 metres free-style, 50 metres backstroke, to tread water for one minute, to float unsupported for five minutes, and so on. If you can do this, and more—excellent. If you can't, try and learn to improve until you can. However, we have to, and do, appreciate that many people who will buy snorkelling gear and use it, are quite poor swimmers. There are no rules to stop them, and provided they are sensible and know their limitations, there is no real harm done. We have, however, to take account of such people in this book, so our third rule is:—

3. **NEVER DO ANYTHING WEARING SNORKELLING EQUIPMENT WHICH YOU CAN'T OR WOULDN'T DO WITHOUT IT.** If you normally never go out of your depth, or swim more than fifty yards from the beach when swimming free, don't do so when snorkelling, however much easier it becomes.
   There are other rules, and they take effect depending on where you dive and how adventurous you are, and we will cover them later. The above rules are **BASIC,** and you ignore them at your peril. If you are fairly healthy, can swim, and are not a complete fool, the time has come to buy some equipment.

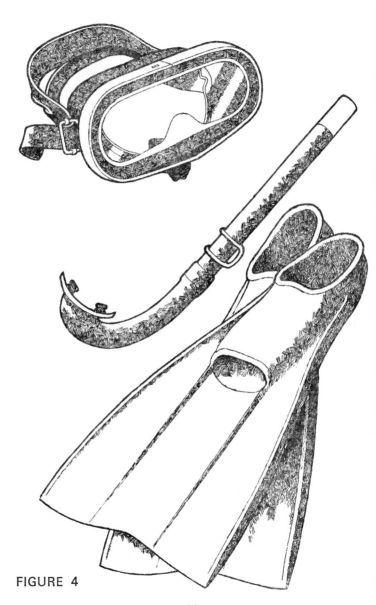

FIGURE 4

Chapter 2

## BUYING EQUIPMENT

Buying equipment is always a problem, for while decent kit is not too expensive, and one can buy all one is likely to need for about £12 ($24) at 1976 prices, the selection is often limited, and decent stockists hard to find.

## WHERE TO BUY

Wherever possible, go to a sports shop, a sub-aqua specialist, or a yacht chandler. They are more likely to have the right gear than a tourist shop selling sun oil and postcards. They may also be able to advise you about local conditions, winds, tides and currents, and such advice is worth having. Remember to ask for it, and pay attention to any sound advice you receive.

## MASKS

The facemask is the most important piece of equipment. Do not buy a mask which incorporates a breathing tube. Mask and tube must be separate.

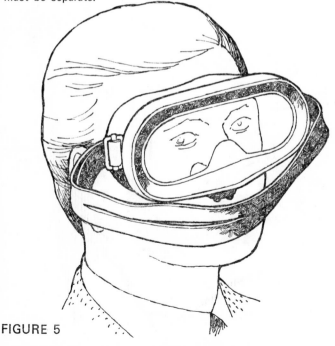

FIGURE 5

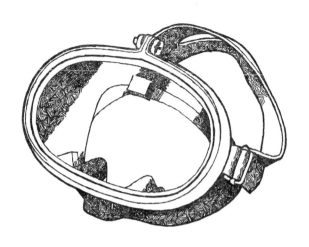

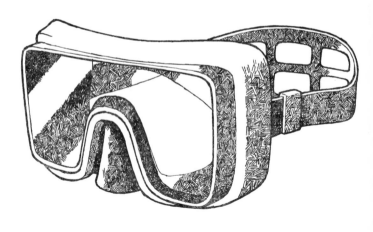

FIGURE 6

The facemask should be of shatterproof glass, not plastic, and made from a good quality synthetic rubber. It should enclose the eyes and nose, but not the mouth, and should be comfortable on the face. The strap must be strong and the buckles secure. See **Fig. 6** for examples of good facemasks.

The mask **must** be airtight, and the test for this is simple. With the strap out of the way and hair pushed back from the forehead, position the mask to your face, enclosing the nose and eyes. Breathe in sharply through the nose, and the mask should be held against the face. Hold your breath and remove your hand. The mask should stay in position, on its own, without support (Fig. 5).

Examine the mask carefully. Inside, just behind the edge, there **ought to be another more shallow lip** of thin flexible rubber. This will serve as an additional seal. Finally, be sure that your mask has a **compensator**, that is, a nose pocket, which allows you to pinch the nostrils and equalize pressure on the ears, and that you **can** pinch your nose through it.

**Facemasks are also available with separate lenses** which can be ground to suit your own prescription, should you wear glasses.

Don't buy goggles, or a simple mask which does not enclose the nose; they have their uses but they are not for you.

Some manufacturers coat their equipment with a silicone shield, to prevent the rubber perishing in store. You will need to clean this coating off the glass of the facemask with a cleaning spirit or petrol. Remember to wash the mask afterwards. If this is not done, vision through the glass may be impaired.

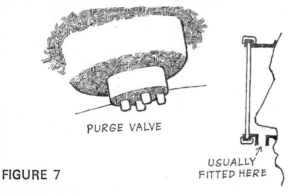

PURGE VALVE

USUALLY
FITTED HERE

**FIGURE 7**

## PURGE VALVES

Some masks, like the one in the illustration, incorporate a purge valve. This is a small drain valve at the lowest point of the mask. Should water leak into the mask, a gentle exhalation through the nose will expel the water, through the purge valve. They are therefore quite useful, but we feel that the best way to clear a flooded mask is by knowing and using the appropriate mask clearing technique which we will teach later on.

Have a purge valve and use it by all means, but don't neglect to learn and practise an essential safety drill as well.

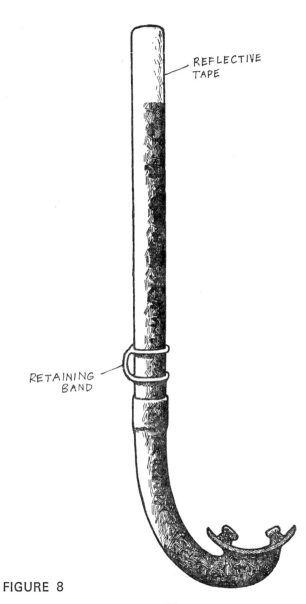

REFLECTIVE
TAPE

RETAINING
BAND

FIGURE 8

18

## SNORKEL TUBES

Don't buy a snorkel tube incorporating any sort of valve, or water excluder at its upper end, be it a cap or a ping-pong ball or whatever. All you need is a plain open-top tube with a mouthpiece. If your tube has such a valve, strip it off, and don't use it. Such valves are of no benefit to the trained snorkel diver, and have sometimes proved dangerous. No experienced aqualung diver uses a valved snorkel tube. People buy valved tubes because they fear water running down the tube and choking them; this doesn't really happen. We will show you how to clear water from a snorkel tube very simply, and there are fewer problems this way than you will encounter with a valve. You may also encounter tubes which have the valve at the lower, mouthpiece end. Avoid these at all costs.

The tube should not be too long, about fifteen inches maximum; made of hard rubber or plastic. The mouthpiece should be of a softer rubber, with moulded pegs to grip with the teeth, and a thin flange which lies between the front teeth and lips. Snorkels may be L or J shaped as in Fig. 8.

The snorkel tube is usually fitted to the left-hand side strap of the facemask by a rubber band or plastic clip, supplied with the snorkel. It is possible to thrust the tube under the mask strap, next to the face, but, it may cause the mask to ease off the face and flood, thereby adding to your problems.

The top of the tube should be bound with a 2'' wide band of red fluorescent tape. This will help you to be more conspicuous on the surface, and is a sensible safety feature.

## FINS

These come in normal shoe sizes, running up to several feet in length for pukka racing fins. You don't need these yet. A normal sized pair, with a blade length equal to your foot length will be just right.

The slipper type is preferable to the heel-strap type, and the fins should be of synthetic rubber, fairly soft for the foot part, but with stiffening ribs at the root. These ribs should taper away to nothing at the tip of the fin, so that it is flexible at the end. If you hold the fin up at eye level, the blade should droop downwards, rather gracefully, in relation to the shoe part (Fig. 9). This droop extends the straight line along the leg which is required to achieve the correct finning action.

The fins should be tried on bare feet, and the fit should be slightly loose rather than too tight. Tight fins lead to cramp. Aim for a comfortable fit, without any pinching across the instep or crushing up of the toes.

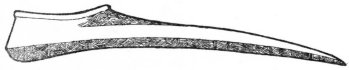

FIGURE 9

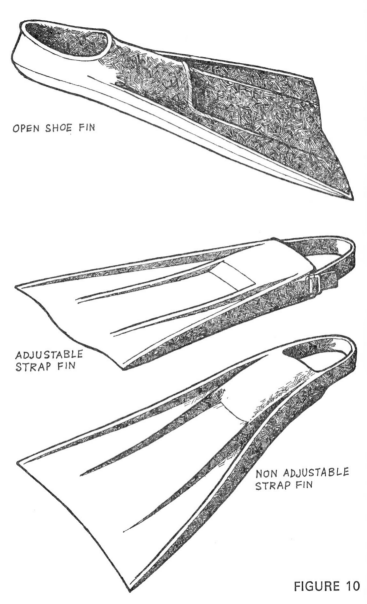

OPEN SHOE FIN

ADJUSTABLE
STRAP FIN

NON ADJUSTABLE
STRAP FIN

FIGURE 10

20

Ill-fitting fins can blister the foot, for the skin gets no chance to harden in the water, but it is difficult to know just how good the fit will be until you try them out in the water. You can, of course, always wear a pair of socks if the fins are a little loose; or prevent chafing with a strip of adhesive tape. Stockists may allow you to return and swap a pair of fins if you find, in practice, that they just don't fit. Ask the shopkeeper if you can do this, and keep the receipt. Fin Retainers (Fig. 11) are available to prevent fins slipping off. They may also prove useful if the fins are slightly too large.

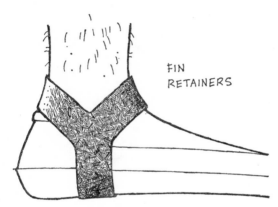

FIN RETAINERS

FIGURE 11

## PRICES

Prices vary with quality and place of purchase. A good mask can cost from £3.50 to £12.00 ($7.00 to $24.00). One costing less than £3.00 ($6.00) would be suspect. Snorkel tubes cost about £1.00 ($2.00). Fins for adults cost from £5.00 ($10.00) upwards, and slightly less for children.

These prices are U.K. and U.S. 1976. Local prices overseas may vary, but since it is important to have good equipment, the lower prices should be taken as minimum; don't buy cheap equipment, whatever you do. Seek advice as to reputable brand names and 'best buys'.

In addition to this basic equipment, if you get keen on the sport, you will soon want or need to acquire other items.

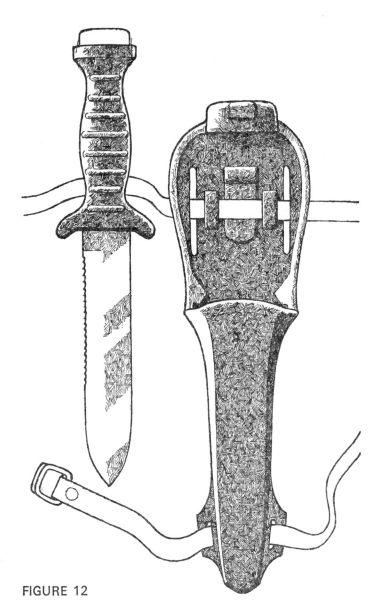

FIGURE 12

## DIVING KNIFE

The rule is that every diver should carry a knife. The problem is that, glancing along any beach, you won't see many snorkellers advancing on the waves with a knife stuck in their sock.

However, let us use commonsense. If you are diving anywhere where you are likely to encounter kelp, ropes, nets or fishing line, a knife is **vital**. Nylon fishing line, which fishermen throw away by the mile, trapping birds and strangling wild life, can entangle you on the bottom. You won't be able to see it, and if you try snapping it, you will cut your hands to the bone. The real answer is for fishermen to take greater care, but as they seem unwilling to consider anyone's affairs but their own, one must take precautions. A typical diving knive is shown in Fig. 12. It should be of robust construction, with a blade length of about 8". One edge of the blade should be serrated; the other a plain knife edge. The handle should have a hilt to prevent the hand slipping on to the blade. Divers' knives are supplied with a leg sheath, so that they may be worn on the calf of the leg. This sheath should have a retaining band which secures the handle when the knife is stowed away. You must be able to reach your knife with either hand. Keep the blade sharp and clean. Remember that a sharp knife can be dangerous, especially to small children and bare feet, so keep it in the sheath and when ashore, stow it away. Knives cost from £5.00 ($10.00) upwards, for a good one.

## WET SUITS

If you get bitten by the snorkelling bug and wish to stay in the water for long periods in all seasons, you will need a wet suit, to keep warm. These come in a variety of sizes, styles and prices. The 'best buy' is a nylon-lined suit, of either smooth or meshed surfaced rubber, costing £20.00 ($40.00) upwards. In cold waters, wet suits are essential; in summer, in warm waters, or for the holiday snorkeller, they are not (Fig. 14).

## LIFE JACKETS

Whenever you go snorkelling in open water, you should wear a life jacket. This should be a fully inflatable jacket, in red or yellow, of B.S.I. standard, inflated by a tug on a carbon dioxide ($CO_2$) cartridge. The deflated life jacket will not add to your diving or swimming problems, but will be a great comfort—a lifesaver in fact—if you get tired or into trouble. Remember to check the $CO_2$ cartridges regularly, and carry a spare in your dive bag.

There are many more gadgets and knick-knacks the enthusiastic snorkeller can purchase. The above are either essential or very useful, and you should buy them as you need them. All instruction in this book is based on the use of the basic items of equipment; mask, fins and snorkel, but remember that as you get more skilled, and more adventurous, you must, for safety's sake, carry or wear the appropriate equipment.

## CARE OF EQUIPMENT

Always sluice down your gear in fresh water after diving. When stowing your gear away for the winter, dust the fins with french chalk, put the equipment in a cool place and avoid crushing it under heavy objects. Hang the wet suit on a padded coat hanger.

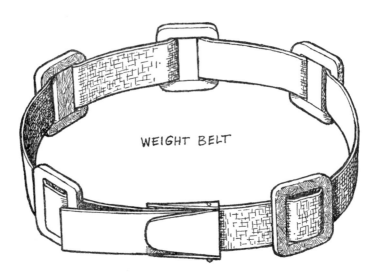

FIGURE 13

## WEIGHT BELT

If you wear a wet suit, and only if you wear a wet suit, you will need a weight belt. Most people are positively buoyant and tend to float rather than sink. The material from which a wet suit is made is inherently buoyant, and to overcome this buoyancy, so that you can dive, the diver must carry weights. These are carried on a strong waist belt, with a quick release buckle (Fig. 13). The trained diver must be able to fasten and unfasten this belt underwater, by feel alone.

The amount of weight needed will depend on your build, and the thickness of the suit. Start with 10 lb. (5 kg.) and use this test to get it right. On breathing in, you should have a tendency to float. When you breath out you should sink beneath the surface. Add or subtract weights until you can control your buoyancy through positive to negative, by depth of breathing.

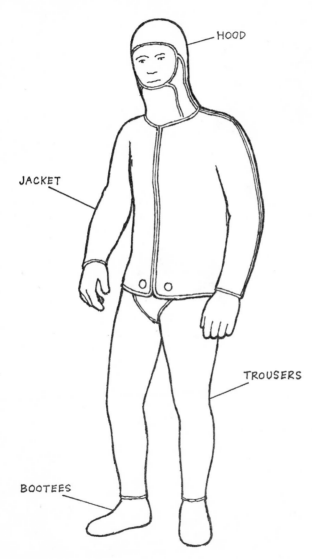

HOOD

JACKET

TROUSERS

BOOTEES

**FIGURE 14**

FIGURE 15

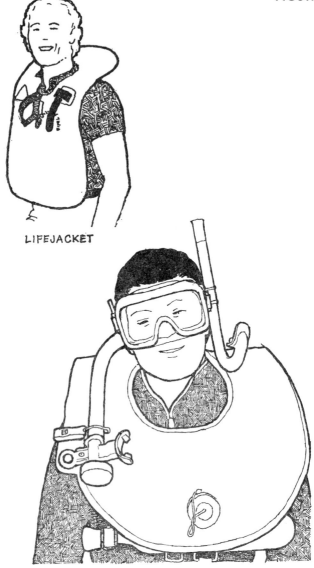

LIFEJACKET

## TRAINING

## WHERE TO TRAIN

The ideal place is an indoor heated swimming pool. Here you have varying depth, useful aids like steps and a handrail, and in warm water you can continue practising for two or three hours without difficulty. Safety is also less of a problem, for if all else fails, in most of the pool you can just stand up!

But most pools do not encourage freelance snorkel swimmers, funnelling such activities into club nights. Hotel pools on holiday are more obliging and you can always learn in shallow offshore waters. For the purposes of this book we will assume that initial training takes place in a swimming pool. Wherever you learn, learn with a friend. Never dive alone. Your pal can assist in the training, and you can coach each other on the finer points of the various drills.

## FITTING EQUIPMENT

Fit the snorkel tube to the left-hand side of the mask strap with the retaining band provided. Place mask, snorkel and flippers on the side of the pool and enter the water.

## ANTI-MISTING

A cold facemask fitted to a warm face will quickly mist up. To prevent this, follow this simple procedure. Spit into the mask. Rub the saliva thoroughly over the inside of the glass and then rinse the mask. It is now ready to put on, and it won't mist up.

## FIT THE MASK

You must keep your hair out of the way. Put the strap over the mask face, and pushing the hair back off the forehead, place the mask in position and breathe in through your nose to hold the mask on to your face. Use both hands to get the strap over and behind the head. Most straps are split in the middle to allow part of it to go above the crown and part under it (Fig. 16).

## FIT THE SNORKEL

Fit the mouthpiece comfortably in the mouth and grip the lugs in the teeth. Have the tube angled back over the left ear. It can be over either ear, of course, but aqualung divers usually have the snorkel on the left side because their demand valve comes over the right side, and you might as well do the same.

## FIT THE FINS

To fit the fins, move into chest-deep water where the water offers support while you are standing on one foot, but remain within reach of the pool side. Slip the toes in, and pull the heel pocket up over the heel. If the slipper fins are tight, you can fold down the back of the heel pocket, push the foot in, and then slip it back up again. Only when you have more experience should you put fins on before entering the water. You can all too easily trip over. When putting fins on before entering the water, wet both feet and fins.

## WALKING IN FLIPPERS

The best way to walk in flippers is to walk backwards! The very shape of the fin blade causes it to bend under your feet as you walk forwards, and you can esily trip over your own feet! So walk backwards, carefully sliding your feet along the bottom.

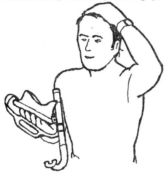

I. PUSH HAIR BACK

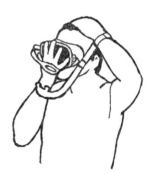

2. PLACE MASK IN POSITION

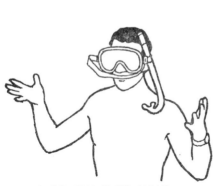

3. BREATH IN TO HOLD MASK ON FACE

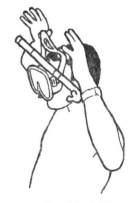

4. EASE STRAP OVER BEHIND THE HEAD

**FIGURE 16**

# Chapter 4

## SNORKEL SWIMMING

With the basic gear fitted dip down in the water to eye level with half the mask covered. Now look at your partner.

You will notice that he appears much wider below the surface than above. This illustrates the distorting effect of vision through water (Fig. 17).

Now hold on to the rail, place your face in the water, and breathe in evenly through the snorkel. Float off, holding on to the side rail and rest in the water, looking down. Get used to breathing through the tube and check that the mask isn't leaking. If it is, check that the edge seal is not tucked in and that no hair is trapped beneath the edge of the mask, allowing water to trickle in.

## CLEARING THE SNORKEL TUBE

Start at the shallow end, so that you can stand up if you need to. Hold on to the pool rail, and float off. Lower the face into the water, and taking a shallow or medium breath, hold it; place the tongue behind the teeth and against the roof of your mouth to seal it off, and submerge about 12" to 18", to arm's length. Keep your eyes open. You will hear the water filling the tube, but with the tongue behind the teeth, it won't enter your mouth.

Stay under until the tube is full—for a count of five—then ease yourself up slowly. As you float back to surface, but keeping the face under, blow *SHARPLY* to force the water out of the tube. It will shoot into the air and shower the spectators. You need the sort of puff that you use to blow out the candles on a birthday cake (Fig. 18)

Now, to do this successfully will take a little bit of practice— say half a dozen goes. Take turns with your partner, each giving the other advice, and you will soon see how to do it.

It may happen that the first blast does not totally clear the tube. You gulp in air and, horrors, you get a mouthful of water. This is why you start at the pool side in shallow water where you can remove the tube, have a good cough, and try again. However, after say, three goes, you won't be so alarmed and then you should try the following. Don't pull out the tube, but tilt your head to one side, the right, snorkel lower-most, keeping the face in the water, and breathe again. Tilting the head gets the little water still in the tube to accumulate at the lowest point, and you can bubble air past it, into your lungs. Another sharp blow will expel the rest of the water, and you are again breathing normally. The secret does lie in giving a good SHARP puff.

To learn tube-clearing will take about ten minutes. You then need a bit of practice and before half an hour is out you will have the knack. There really is no more to it, and this done, you can start finning.

**FIGURE 17**

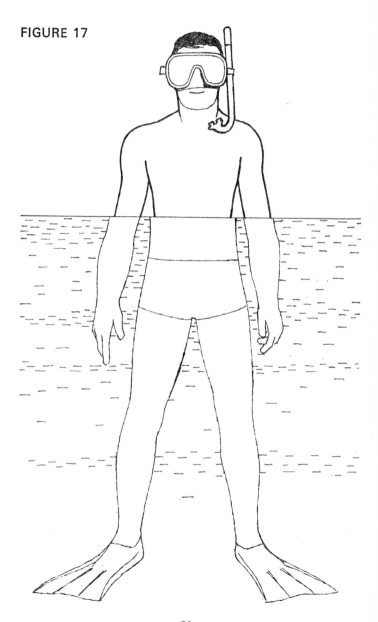

FIGURE 18

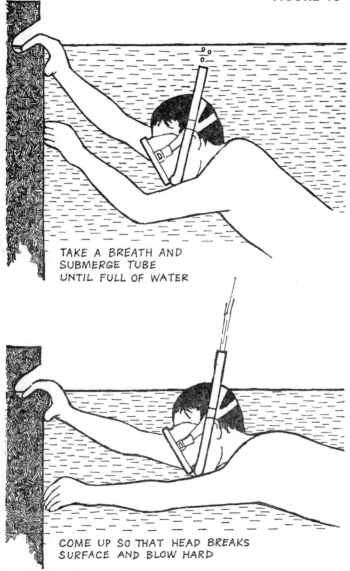

TAKE A BREATH AND
SUBMERGE TUBE
UNTIL FULL OF WATER

COME UP SO THAT HEAD BREAKS
SURFACE AND BLOW HARD

## FINNING ACTION

Holding on to the side of the pool in the shallow end again, lower your face into the water; float off at arm's length, and breathing through your snorkel, gently practise the finning action (Fig. 19).

This action can take a deal of practise to learn correctly, so pay attention to the following points:

1   Look ahead—watch where you are going. If you want to look down, stop finning. Keeping the face forward also helps the body position.

2   **The legs should lie angled down at about 10°-15°, not flailing** on the surface.

3   The action is a horizontal scissors stride, from the hips, NOT a pedalling action from the knee.

4   Initially, concentrate on keeping the knees straight. You will have to bend them a little, but by trying to keep them straight you help to get the correct finning action. Study the diagrams (Figs. 20 and 21). The first diagram shows the correct position in the water; the second shows the correct finning action.

Once you feel reasonably sure that you have the basics, try a few gentle trips to and fro across the pool. No diving yet. Just concentrate on finning and breathing. Keep the fins submerged and do not use the arms at all; keep them at your sides or link your thumbs behind your back (Fig. 20).

Don't try and go too fast, and aim for an even stroke. Look ahead at an angle of 45°. If you want to study the bottom, stop. Concentrate on developing a good action. You will swim a long way when snorkelling, and a poor style is tiring. Common faults are (a) Not keeping the toes pointed down; (b) Fluttering from the knees with minimal hip movement; (c) Fins breaking the surface because your 'seat' is too high in the water. Look at Fig. . . . . again.

## TREADING WATER

Every swimmer should be able to tread water. With the extra power fins impart, it is easily done. The snorkeller needs to acquire this skill so that he may adjust or replace his mask and tube, to have a look round, or just to chat to his partner.

Go deeper into the pool, so that you are out of your depth, holding the rail to one side if you prefer, and let the legs down; Start a striding action with the legs, with the toes pointing down; at the same time keep your balance with to-and-fro hand movements under the surface. You will find it easy to maintain yourself at shoulder level. To resume swimming, simply lean forward and fin away face down.

Now increase the beat with the legs, and the fins will power you up out of the water, chest high. You can use this movement for a good look round, or to start a dive, as we will show in the next chapter.

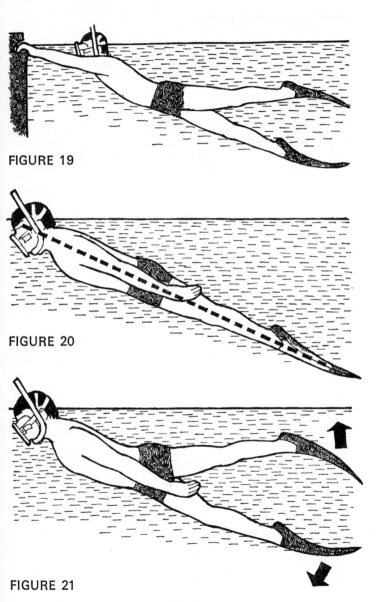

FIGURE 19

FIGURE 20

FIGURE 21

## FINNING ON YOUR BACK

A variation to the normal face down finning position, is to fin lying on your back. The snorkel should be removed, and you breathe through your mouth. It is easy to move into this method from a treading water position. Simply lean back, as you tread water and, hey presto!—you are finning on your back.

## FINNING VARIATIONS

*Dolphin Kicks and Side Swimming:* Two other methods of finning can be employed to help you along and give you a rest from the normal finning action. Underwater you can employ the Dolphin kick, beating with *both* legs and fins together. On the surface you can roll onto your side, snorkel uppermost, and fin along on your side. It makes a change and can be used to rest your muscles.

Chapter 5

# SNORKEL DIVING

Having mastered the basic skills of tube clearing, finning and treading water, you are now ready to start getting, and briefly staying, under water. You need to be able to submerge with the minimum of wasted effort, and a clean, well executed Jack-Knife Dive is the best way. But first, a word about breathing.

## BREATHING

In snorkelling, as in most active sports, correct breathing is crucial. The big error is to take too big a breath. A deep breath increases your buoyancy, making it harder to dive, and is harder to hold. You feel your lungs are bursting. Keep your breathing normal, regular and controlled. Before diving take a couple of deep breaths, then a normal relaxed breath to take with you when you dive. Hold that breath until you return to the surface.

## HYPERVENTILATION AND ANOXIA

Hyperventilation is the word employed to describe deep, rapid breathing prior to a breath-held dive. The object is to remove carbon-dioxide and saturate the lungs and body with oxygen, and enable the diver to stay down longer. There is no hard evidence that hyperventilation increases diving times, which are improved far more by correct techniques and economy of effort. There is, however, plenty of evidence that hyperventilation is dangerous, for it can lead to **Anoxia**. Anoxia is a condition normally caused by lack of oxygen in the blood, which rapidly affects the brain and leads to unconsciousness.

Hyperventilation is dangerous because it reduces the level of carbon dioxide in the blood, and this can be fatal, for it is the rising concentration of $CO_2$ in the blood as the oxygen is consumed that triggers the impulse to draw the next breath. Breathing is an automatic reaction and we usually do it without being aware of it. Hyperventilation increases the oxygen in the blood and lowers the $CO_2$ level. During the dive, the $CO_2$ in the blood builds up towards its normal level, but the oxygen is used up before the $CO_2$ level reaches the point necessary to trigger the desire for another breath, and the diver loses consciousness and, if underwater, drowns. This process happens very quickly and totally without warning, and death is the usual result. Never employ hyperventilation before a dive. Take no more than two good breaths before diving, and don't stay down once you feel the first urge to come up. Always dive in pairs, and have one person on the surface, watching, while the other dives.

A diver can be affected by Anoxia during an ascent or after surfacing. He will be making strong breathing efforts and will be blue about the lips, finger nails and ear lobes. It may be necessary to apply mouth to mouth resuscitation, and get the victim quickly to hospital. There is no self-help for anoxia.

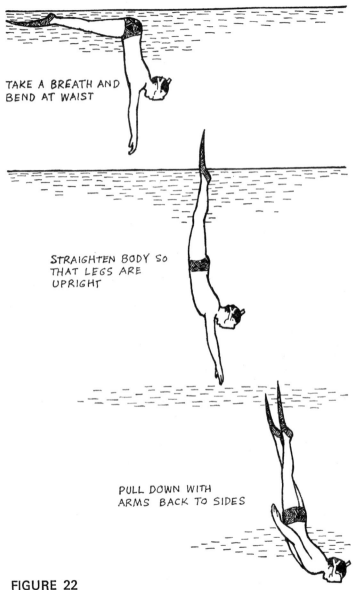

TAKE A BREATH AND
BEND AT WAIST

STRAIGHTEN BODY SO
THAT LEGS ARE
UPRIGHT

PULL DOWN WITH
ARMS BACK TO SIDES

**FIGURE 22**

36

## JACK-KNIFE DIVING

To practise this, swim to-and-fro across the pool in about shoulder deep water. Then you can stand up if you have to. Swim along, in the surface finning position, and prepare to dive.

Take a normal breath; bend forward from the waist so that the trunk of your body is pointing downward under the surface. At the same time, give one breast stroke, pull with the arms, to pull the body under, and lift the legs straight up in the air above you. The fins should come over your head, well out of the water. The weight of your legs will push you easily to the bottom (Fig.22). The drill then is:

1   Breathe in.

2   Bend and pull the body under.

3   Legs up and together,—dive!

At shoulder depth or in shallower water, you will need to dive at an angle, 'pulling out' before you hit the bottom of the pool! In deeper water you can start by going down almost vertically, using your downward weight to propel you along. Don't dive down and crumple up in a heap on the bottom. Start finning only when you are well and truly underwater. Level out from the dive, and fin on for a few yards before surfacing. Apart from the initial breast stroke pull, don't use the arms at all. Remember to clear your ears if discomfort is felt at depth, and if the mask appears to be pressing hard against your face, exhale air into it through your nose to prevent mask squeeze.

## SURFACING

When surfacing come up with the head back, looking up at the surface. This is a safety drill, and is best learnt to begin with. You don't want to surface under an obstruction, or butt another swimmer in the middle, so look up, ascend, and as your head breaks surface, blast the water out of your snorkel tube, and have a quick look round before you fall back to the surface, face down, to catch your breath again. Safety drills must be used wherever and whenever you practise, until they are second nature. In the open water situation, you might surface in the path of a boat or in some other hazardous situation. Look up and look around (Fig. 23).

Practise this dive, the basic snorkel dive, in pairs or threesomes, with one person always watching from the surface. It's quite exciting and you can correct each other's mistakes, treading water for a natter after every few dives. Practise this until you are, in your own and your partner's opinion, diving neatly and have every confidence in clearing the tube on surfacing. Then move on to deeper waters, and practise until you are crossing the pool underwater on one breath, and swimming the length of the pool underwater on two breaths. Let your progress in diving be natural rather than forced. Just keep practising and the improvements will follow. If it doesn't feel right, it probably isn't.

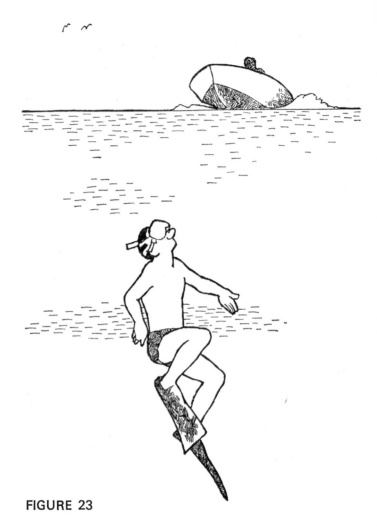

FIGURE 23

## FEET FIRST DIVE

The feet first dive comes from the treading water position. Tread water hard to drive the body up out of the water, pushing down with the outstretched arms at the same time. As your arms reach your hips, stop treading, breathe in, and the weight of your now rigid, vertical body will push you well below the surface, where you bend forward and fin away (Fig. 24).

## FORWARD AND BACKWARD ROLLS

At this stage of training you need to concentrate on improving your underwater skills and control. One way of doing this is by practising underwater rolls.

## FORWARD ROLLS

(Fig. 25) Go into a forward roll underwater by continuing the Jack-Knife dive. This goes, as you will recall; body under; breast stroke; legs up; dive.

As you dive, curl the body forward, drawing the legs up to the chest. Scoop the water evenly with outstretched arms to keep the body rolling forward in this tucked position.

## BACKWARD ROLLS

Start this from the surface by finning along on your back; breathe; arch the back, and with hands and arms in the water above your head, push the water away from you. This will carry you under into a backward roll.

Do not fin at all, let the legs trail limply behind you as you rotate yourself evenly by sweeping the arms forward, as if pushing the water away from you. You can turn head-over-heels several times like this, before you surface.

Underwater rolls are of little practical application, but they are very useful for increasing confidence and control underwater, and above all, they are good fun!

Having gone this far, the secret is practise, practise, and more practise, until you feed completely at ease at diving, rolling, swimming on the surface and clearing the tube.

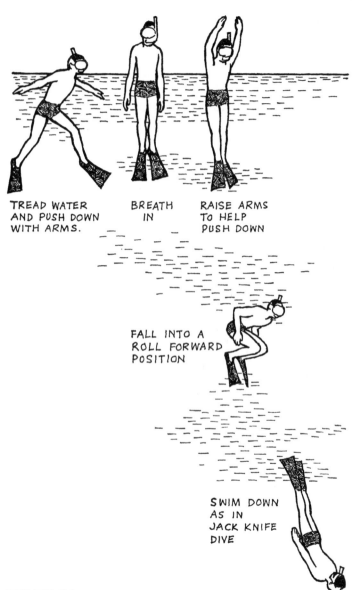

TREAD WATER AND PUSH DOWN WITH ARMS.

BREATH IN

RAISE ARMS TO HELP PUSH DOWN

FALL INTO A ROLL FORWARD POSITION

SWIM DOWN AS IN JACK KNIFE DIVE

**FIGURE 24**

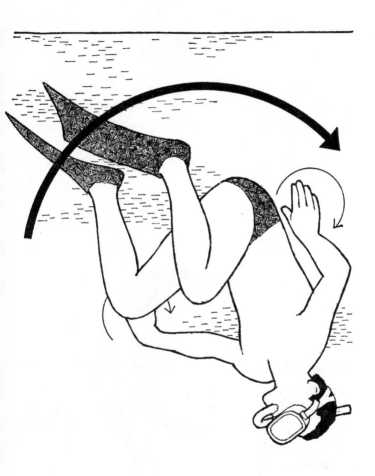

FIGURE 25

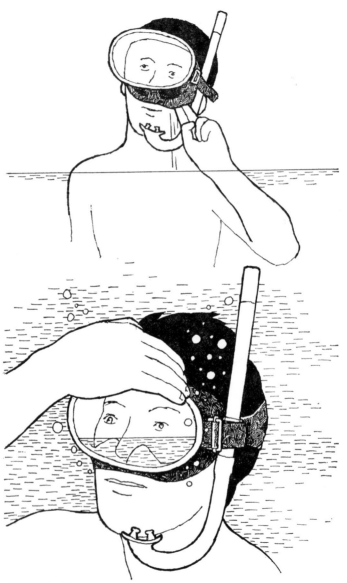

FIGURE 26

# Chapter 6

## PROBLEMS

Once you are confident that you know what to do when things go well, **we** can proceed to practise a few drills for accidents or emergencies. Nothing drastic, you understand, just learning to cope with those little run-of-the-mill difficulties. The first of these is a flooded facemask.

## CLEARING THE FACEMASK

In shallow water, if you flood the mask completely, the drill is to surface, tread water, and lift the lower edge of the mask to allow the water to drain away. Don't remove the mask completely.

Even if your mask has a purge valve, you should know how to clear it by the fundamental method of displacing water with air. Once learnt the drill is quite easy, but it does need practice, and you should practise flooding and clearing your mask every time you go snorkelling. It is also good training and a confidence drill, to learn how to clear the mask while underwater, by blowing air into the mask from the nose. Practise this as follows: Go shoulder-deep in the water, breathe, duck under and flood the mask by easing the *upper* edge off the forehead. To clear, while still underwater tilt the head back and *press* on the upper edge of the mask. This eases the *bottom* edge away from the face. As you do this, exhale steadily through the nose. This will force the water out of the bottom of the mask and when it is clear, take your hand off the top rim. Practise this a few times until you have the drill right. Even if you only half clear the mask you can breathe in through the tube, float vertically with head back, and exhale again to finish the job. The water must be at the bottom of the mask, not swilling about against the glass, so head back, remember. This drill takes a fair amount of practice, but you should be able to master the basics in about half-an-hour (Fig. 26).

## MASK SQUEEZE

The mask has to be airtight and on a deeper dive it can happen that the pressure squeezes the mask hard against the face. In extreme cases this can result in black or bloodshot eyes. This pressure must be equalised by snorting air down the nostrils into the mask. (See introduction.)

## LOST EQUIPMENT

You can and will, from time to time, lose your equipment. Often, when jumping into the water, your facemask can be dislodged, or the water can wash a fin off. You must therefore be able to recover them.

## LOST FACEMASK AND TUBE

Try and watch where they fall. Without a mask you will have difficulty seeing them underwater, but once they are located, jack-knife dive down and pick them up. On surfacing, look round and if all is clear, tread water. Then replace mask as taught on page 27. Remember to keep the hair out of the way. If there is still water in the mask, clear it by draining out the water from the bottom rim. Replace snorkel in your mouth and blow clear.

## LOST MASK, TUBE AND FINS

When you have lost the lot you should first try and recover the fins. For mobility underwater, and for treading water, they are essential; and as they are both large and black, they are easy to find. Pick the fins up and return to the surface, holding them by the heels. Held any other way they provide a surprising amount of resistance to surfacing. You may prefer to pick them up one at a time, as this way it is easier to fit them on, even if it means more dives. When fitting fins in the water, take a breath and duck your face under, bringing the foot up as you bend your body down. Don't try to put the fin on while keeping your face above water.

Once you have your fins on you can go through the mask and tube drill as shown above.

## LOST WEIGHT BELT

The word 'lost' is really for convenience. You may need to jettison your weight belt quite deliberately for a number of reasons, leaving the weights on the bottom. Practising this in a pool, don't let the weights crash on the bottom. Broken pool tiles are expensive!

Weight belts are also expensive, so you will want to recover it. When doing this you must be totally relaxed, and not out of breath. Once located, dive down to the belt, and holding one end, turn round to sit on the bottom. Reach for the other end and pulling the ends together around your body, clip the belt back on. Give a good kick off the bottom at the start of your ascent.

This, as with everything else takes practice, but it is much easier to refit the belt on the bottom, than to do so while swimming along or while treading water. You don't have to hold it up, just for a start! Try it and you will see. This drill assumes, of course, that the weight belt has fallen in a depth and place where you can safely reach it. Better buy a new belt rather than take unnecessary risks.

Finally, remember that you are always doing this with a partner, never alone. If you lose your mask and visibility is poor, he can dive and get it for you, and you can do the same for him sometime. That's what friends are for.

# Chapter 7

## ENTERING THE WATER

Up to now we have assumed that you have gone down a ladder, or waded into the water.

You should also learn some other ways of getting in, but remember at this point another basic rule, "NEVER GET IN UNLESS YOU CAN GET OUT".

## STRIDE ENTRY

The simplest way to enter from a low bank or pier, is the stride entry, (Fig. 27). As the name indicates, you simply stand up, hold mask and snorkel in position, using both hands, and take a good long stride away from the side, entering the water with legs apart to break your fall. From anything other than a low height, say three feet, this can sometimes be a trifle painful—especially for men! Watch the height carefully.

## ROLLS

The other basic entries are forward and backward rolls, and a vertical jump; the two former from heights of up to two feet above the water, and the latter from heights over this, up to twenty feet.

The idea is to enter the water easily, and fully equipped, without the rush of water stripping off mask and snorkel, if not the flippers.

Fig. 28 shows the entry positions for the forward and backward rolls. In each case the diver squats or sits on the very edge of the jetty or boat and rolls into the water, holding mask and snorkel FIRMLY against the face, and aiming to land on the shoulders.

It is not sufficient just to place your hands over the face mask, for the water impact is considerable. You must hold the mask firmly in position until your entry is complete.

## VERTICAL ENTRY

The vertical entry emphasises the problems of retaining mask and flippers. The starting position is as shown in Fig. 29. Note the position of the feet. The fins are overlapped to minimise the water resistance on impact. You would use this for entering the water from a height in excess of about 3 ft., say from the deck of a yacht or cabin cruiser, or from a quay or pier. Remember that water can get very hard indeed over about twelve feet, and aim for a vertical entry, hopping off the side to plunge, arrow-like, into the water. Do not allow the body to lean forward.

Two other forms of entry are the racing dive, and the silent entry. You would use the racing dive to enter from a bank or rock, into shallow water. Holding the mask firmly, you dive in, turning in the air to land on your side, leading with the point of the shoulder. The impact can be considerable. You *must* turn on to your side—never dive in head first.

FIGURE 27

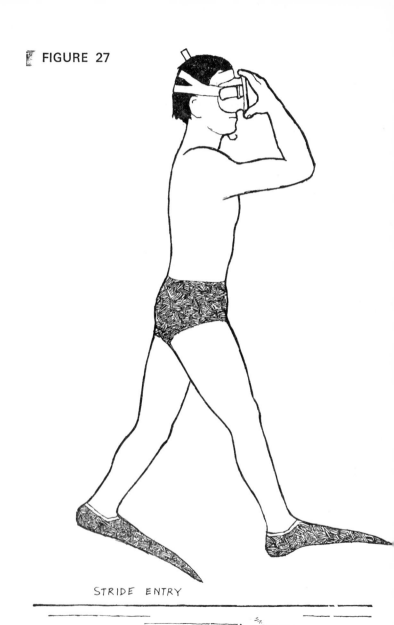

STRIDE ENTRY

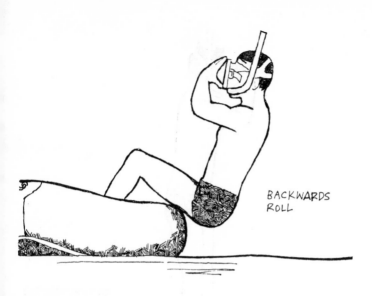

BACKWARDS ROLL

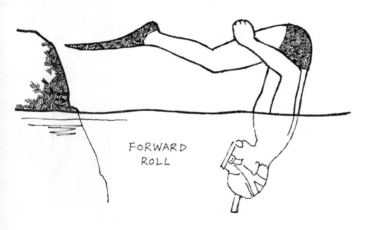

FORWARD ROLL

FIGURE 28

47

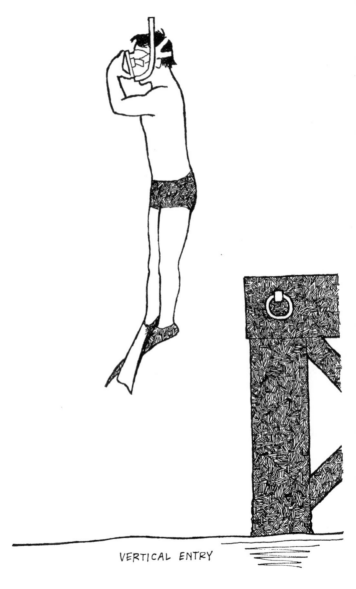

VERTICAL ENTRY

**FIGURE 29**

Occasionally the diver will want to slip quietly into the water, perhaps to avoid scaring fish nearby. The diver sits on the edge, fins in the water, and turning the body, places the hands on the bank, fingers inward, and then slips quietly into the water, supporting the body by the hands, until fully immersed. This can be done without any splashing or disturbance (Fig. 30).

Finally, however you enter the water, check and be sure that you are not jumping or diving on to an obstruction. Check first and be careful.

## LEAVING THE WATER

Never get in unless you can get out. The problems of getting out of the water affect all who enter it, deliberately or accidentally. Anyone who has tried to bring a man-overboard back on to a dinghy, can tell you that.

It is important to leave the water before you are too cold or tired to make the effort. You must also make preparations to leave the water, before you enter.

Wave action over rocks can dash the diver about considerably, and boarding a boat without a ladder is also difficult. Luckily the fins, as we have seen while treading water, can be used to propel the body up, and make the exit easier. If returning to a small boat, climb in by lifting yourself with your arms, as you would when emerging from the deep end of a swimming pool. A bowline tied in a rope, can give support for a foot and help the swimmer climb aboard a larger boat. Every entry situation must be assessed with reference to subsequent exit. Bear that in mind and you won't go far wrong.

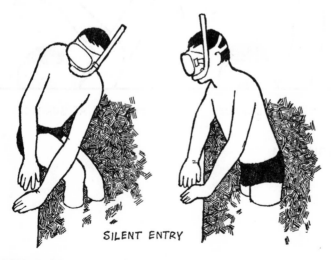

SILENT ENTRY

FIGURE 30

## Chapter 8

## UNDERWATER SIGNALS

Remembering that you never dive alone, but always with a partner, you will, from time to time, want to communicate with each other, both on and under the surface. You can, of course, when on the surface, tread water and chat, but frequently while diving, one will spot something that one wants to show to one's partner. You will also want to let your friends on shore know that you are O.K., or otherwise. The following hand signals are in common use among divers, and should be adopted and used by all new snorkel divers.

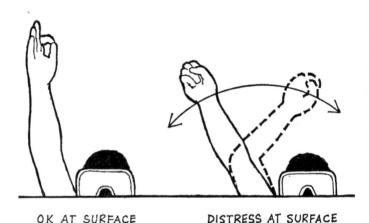

OK AT SURFACE          DISTRESS AT SURFACE

FIGURE 31

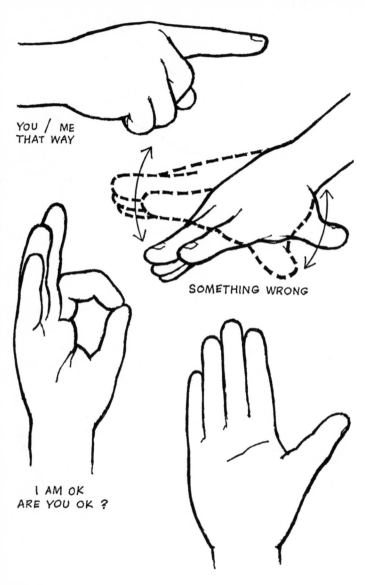

YOU / ME
THAT WAY

SOMETHING WRONG

I AM OK
ARE YOU OK ?

STOP / STAY THERE

FIGURE 32

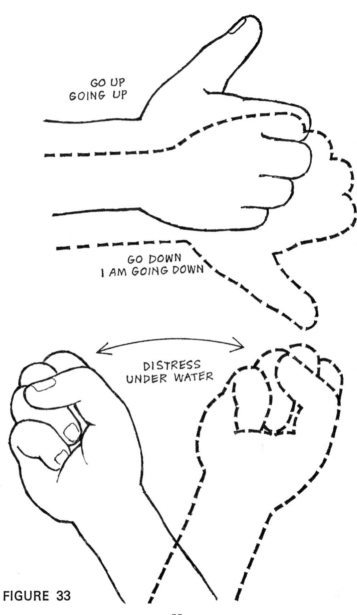

GO UP
GOING UP

GO DOWN
I AM GOING DOWN

DISTRESS
UNDER WATER

FIGURE 33

# Chapter 9

## RESCUE AND RESUSCITATION

Since, even in the best organised affairs, accidents can happen, you must learn and practise established techniques for rescue and resuscitation, both in the water and ashore. The best technique is prevention, by not getting into trouble in the first place. The next best is to have taken adequate precautions so that you can cope with an emergency if it arises. Prevention and precautions are the first two stages to safety, and most of the steps have been mentioned already in this book, but we will, just to be on the safe side, summarise them here:—

## PREVENTION

Buy good equipment, and be well trained in its use. Be able to swim. Never dive alone. Never get in unless you can get out. Come out before you are cold and overtired. Be sensible and *use* your commonsense.

## PRECAUTIONS

Never dive with a cold. Never dive just after a heavy meal. Beware of cold and cramp. In open water wear a wet-suit and life-jacket and have floating support ready. Carry a knife. Get good local information on tides and currents. Practise safety drills regularly.

Now, if you know and apply all this you should be safe, but accidents still occur. Perhaps the person you have to rescue is a stranger—or someone near and dear to you. You must therefore know rescue techniques and expired air resuscitation (mouth to nose) and the more familiar mouth to mouth resuscitation.

## PUSHING AND TOWING

with a tow or a push. For the co-operative diver, a push is probably the best. For this the pusher grasps the tired diver's If your partner gets tired and needs help, you can help him greatly wrists and, holding them together by twisting the palms of the subject's hands uppermost, pushes him towards the shore (Fig. 34). The subject, on his back, can push up his mask and dispense with his snorkel. This method is very easy to learn, and is not too tiring on the 'rescuer', but does require a conscious and co-operative person in the part of the 'rescued'.

The second method is more suitable for use with an unconscious or struggling diver.

First remove the subject's facemask and snorkel. The rescuer grasps the subject's right armpit with his right hand, thumb forward. He then clamps the subject's left arm against his own chest with his right elbow. The rescuer's left arm goes behind the subject's head to support it, the left hand gripping the victim's left armpit or clothing near the upper arm; rather like getting the subject into a 'half nelson' hold (Fig. 35).

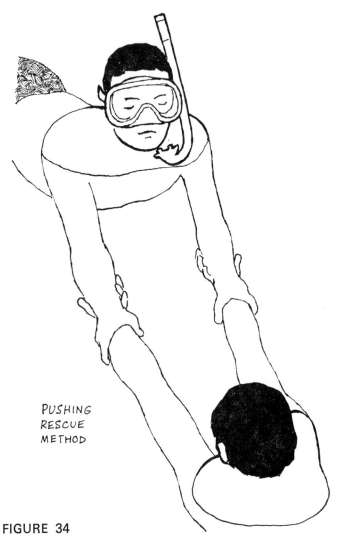

PUSHING
RESCUE
METHOD

FIGURE 34

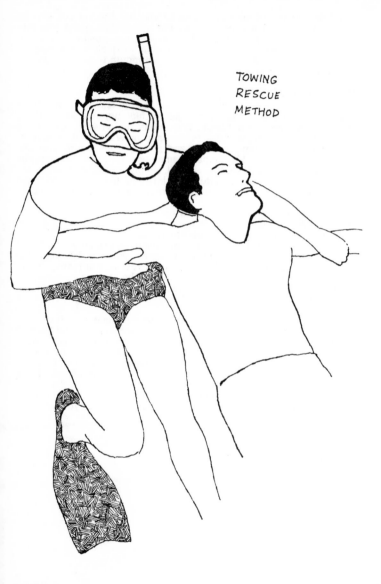

TOWING
RESCUE
METHOD

**FIGURE 35**

Obviously the rescuer will have to spit his snorkel out, but he should keep his mask on in case the subject struggles free and has to be recovered. He is then in a good position to swim backwards, towing his partner, and able to quell any struggles, while keeping his head above water. Give mouth to nose resuscitation if necessary (Fig. 36).

## RESUSCITATION

Once ashore, proceed with mouth to mouth resuscitation. Place the unconscious diver flat on the ground face up, and lift the neck, allowing the head to fall back. This opens the airways. Check the mouth for obstructions, false teeth, sand or weed, and remove it. Then pinch the victim's nostrils, and placing your mouth over his, exhale deeply into his lungs. Remember to keep the nostrils pinched shut, otherwise the air will simply circulate through the airways and out again, instead of inflating the lungs. Continue expired air resuscitation at normal breathing rate, until the victim resumes breathing.

The victim may vomit. Roll him on to his side so that it drains away. Clear his mouth and resume resuscitation. Send for a doctor or medical help at the first opportunity.

Many people quail at the idea of giving resuscitation, but rest assured that when and if the time comes, you will be very glad you know the drill. Learn the methods of rescue and resuscitation, and be sure your partner does so as well. The life he saves may be yours. Do not practise mouth to mouth resuscitation on your boy/girl friend. Breathing into the lungs of a breathing person is dangerous.

Finally, think carefully about going to a rescue if you do not have the skill or strength. The graveyards are full of good-hearted people who were drowned trying to rescue people who were eventually saved by somebody else—or saved themselves. It helps nobody to have two people struggling in the water. Never refuse help in a rescue. We have given methods suitable for a single rescuer, but if you are swimming in a party, get the others to help, even in a simple, helpful tow. Rescuing or helping other swimmers is a very tiring business. Practise it and you will find out yourself.

KEEP
VICTIM'S
MOUTH
CLOSED

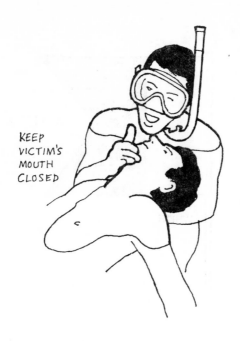

BREATH
INTO
VICTIM'S
NOSE

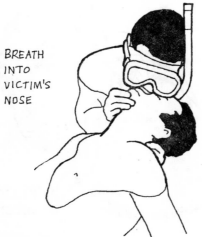

FIGURE 36

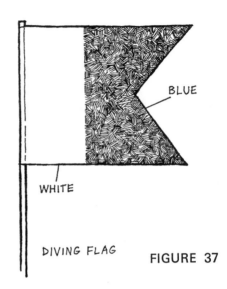

BLUE

WHITE

DIVING FLAG

**FIGURE 37**

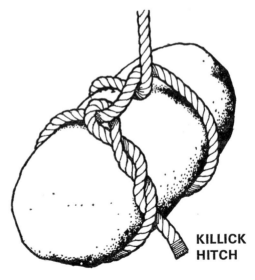

**KILLICK HITCH**

**FIGURE 38**

# Chapter 10

## SWIMMING OFF-SHORE

We stated on page 13, as a basic safety rule, that you should do nothing while wearing a snorkel that you would not do without one. This for the moderate swimmer, is necessarily a limiting factor, for he will soon want to swim further out, drawn invisibly by the greater attractions to be found away from the shoreline, and among off-lying rocks.

To do this and remain inside a safety limit, you must take a support of some sort with you; a rubber raft, or dinghy, or an inflated truck innertube. This you can anchor or moor in the diving area, so that, if you feel tired, or flood your mask, you have something within reach to support you.

If you have a boat or rubber dinghy, one diver should always remain aboard, to assist the swimmers in the water if necessary. The rule is always: one diving, one on the surface. The ratios can vary, but having someone on watch is essential. Having a float on the surface also helps to warn speedboats or water skiers of the presence of divers, especially if the boat carries the official diving flag (Fig. 37).

## CURRENTS AND TIDES

Don't go diving off-shore, in rivers or estuaries, without checking first with local people, fishermen, harbour-masters, or the local sub-aqua club, about prevailing conditions, currents and tide rips. If there is a current, moor your raft on the down-current side of your diving area, swimming up-current to reach your objective. In this way, when you are tired or in trouble, you will not have the current to fight while rejoining the raft.

## MOORING AND ANCHORING

It follows from this that the current must not be permitted to carry the raft away, and it must therefore lie securely moored. If you are diving off a motor boat, yacht or large boat, you will probably have an anchor. This should be put over the side, using *three times* as much anchor cable as there is depth of water under the boat. Smaller dinghies, rubber floats and so on, may not have an anchor, but use can be made of a large stone, secured to the line with a killick hitch (Fig. 38). This hitch will hold the stone firmly, and keep the boat or float in position, and suitable large stones are easy to find.

# Chapter 11

## FURTHER ACTIVITIES

In common with the activities in the other Venture Guides, Snorkelling is as much a means to an end as an end in itself. The knowledge of snorkelling techniques which this book (and practice) will have given you, will extend your appreciation and awareness of a whole new underwater world, and put another range of activities into your grasp.

Most of the sea's teeming marine life is found in the shallower waters within reach of the experienced snorkel diver. The identification of marine species is itself a fascinating pursuit. With care, wrecks lying in shallow water can be explored, and the availability of amphibious cameras gives the photographer the opportunity to extend his horizons below the sea's surface.

Spear-fishing is a dwindling interest as more divers turn towards underwater photography and the study of marine life, and grow more conscious of the need to conserve. However, those who wish to hunt, take up a very challenging pastime, which takes a great deal of time to master. If you want to take up spear-fishing, first study one of the specialist books on the subject. In careless or inexperienced hands, a speargun can be lethal.

Crabs and lobsters may be taken by hand, but don't be greedy. Pot fishermen, whose livelihood depends on these creatures, do not take too kindly to divers taking them. In many countries, the taking of such crustacea by divers is prohibited.

You may wish to progress to aqualung diving. This cannot be carried out safely alone. Sound instruction is vital, and the best instruction is gained through a good diving club or school. In Great Britain, the British Sub Aqua Club is the governing body for the sport, and has a membership of some 30,000 through its 700 branches. All age groups and interests are catered for. The BSAC National Snorkellers Club exists to encourage youngsters (8 to 15 years) to go snorkelling safely. The BSAC Schools and Youth Section introduces teenagers to both snorkelling and aqualung diving, and the Club's branches are open to the adult public who want to try the sport. Instruction in snorkelling and aqualung diving is given at Branch level, and subscription rates are very reasonable. BSAC also has a number of branches overseas, and is the largest single diving club in the world. Why not find out more about BSAC by writing to the Club's headquarters at 70 Brompton Road, London, SW3 1HA.

Other countries outside the U.K. and Commonwealth also have sub-aqua clubs and training centres, and associations. Find out about them from local dive shops, wherever you are, in Spain, Australia, the U.S. or wherever.

For aqualung diving do join a club and receive proper instruction.

Never buy a lung and leap into the nearest water unsupervised. You may never come up!

With snorkel gear, you will have a new world at your flippers, and we hope this look will help you enjoy it.